ESSENTIAL GUIDE TO ECZEMA

Comprehensive Insights and Practical Strategies for Managing and Healing Skin Conditions

DR. CASEY LOREN

DISCLAIMER

This book's content is only meant to be used for general informative purposes. Although the author has taken great care to ensure the content is accurate and thorough, no warranties or assurances on the information's accuracy, correctness, or reliability are provided. It is recommended that readers employ their own judgment and discretion when applying any material found in this book to their particular situation.

The information in this book is not intended to replace professional advice, nor is the author an expert in any of the subjects covered. It is recommended that readers consult with experienced professionals regarding any particular issues or concerns.

Any name that may be mentioned or referred in this book does not imply endorsement, recommendation, or relationship on the part of the author with any person, entity, good, website, or association. These references are made only for informational purposes and are not meant to be taken as recommendations or endorsements.

The information contained in this book may cause readers to suffer loss or damage, for which the author disclaims all obligation and accountability. The only people accountable for the decisions and actions taken by readers using the information presented are themselves.

Any names, characters, companies, locations, activities, occasions, and incidents referenced in this book are either made up or the result of the author's imagination. Any likeness to real people, living or dead, or to real things is entirely coincidental.

This book's content may change at any time, without prior notice, according to the author.

The onus is on the reader to verify whether there have been any updates or revisions.

The reader accepts the conditions of this disclaimer by reading this book. Please do not read this book or use its contents if you do not agree to these terms.

Table of Contents

CHAPTER 1

UNDERSTANDING ECZEMA

Definition and Types of Eczema

Eczema, also known as atopic dermatitis, is a chronic skin condition characterized by inflammation, itchiness, and redness of the skin. It often manifests in patches, which can be dry, scaly, or oozing. There are several types of eczema, each with its distinct characteristics:

1. **Atopic Dermatitis:** This is the most common type, often seen in individuals with a family history of allergic conditions like asthma or hay fever. It typically appears in childhood and may improve with age.

2. **Contact Dermatitis:** This type occurs when the skin comes into contact with irritants or allergens, leading to redness, itching, and sometimes blistering.

3. **Nummular Eczema:** This form of eczema is characterized by coin-shaped patches of irritated skin, which can be very itchy and may ooze fluid.

4. **Dyshidrotic Eczema:** This type affects the palms of the hands, sides of the fingers, and soles of the feet, causing small blisters and intense itching.

5. **Seborrheic Dermatitis:** While not always classified as eczema, seborrheic dermatitis shares similarities with eczema in terms of redness, flaking, and itchiness, commonly affecting the scalp (dandruff), face, and other oily areas of the skin.

Causes and Triggers

The exact cause of eczema is not fully understood, but it is believed to be a combination of genetic and environmental factors. People with eczema often have a compromised skin barrier, making their skin more susceptible to irritation and allergens. Common triggers include:

- **Allergens:** Such as pollen, pet dander, dust mites, and certain foods.

- **Irritants:** Including soaps, detergents, perfumes, and harsh fabrics.

- **Climate:** Dry or humid weather can exacerbate symptoms.

- **Stress:** Emotional stress can trigger or worsen eczema flare-ups.

- **Microbes:** Bacteria, fungi, and viruses can contribute to inflammation.

Symptoms and Signs

The symptoms of eczema can vary depending on the type and severity but often include:

- Intense itching, especially at night

- Dry, scaly, or thickened skin

- Redness and inflammation

- Small, fluid-filled blisters

- Crusting and oozing (in severe cases)

- Darkening or lightening of the skin (after prolonged scratching or healing)

Diagnosing Eczema

Diagnosing eczema typically involves a thorough examination of the skin, a medical history review, and sometimes allergy testing to identify triggers. A dermatologist or allergist can provide a definitive diagnosis and recommend appropriate treatment based on the individual's symptoms and triggers.

Impact on Mental Health

Living with eczema can have a significant impact on mental health. The chronic itching, discomfort, and visible nature of the condition can lead to:

- Anxiety and stress

- Depression

- Sleep disturbances

- Social withdrawal

- Reduced self-esteem and body image issues

Individuals with eczema need to address not only the physical symptoms but also the emotional and psychological aspects through support groups, counseling, and self-care strategies.

Eczema in Children vs. Adults

While eczema can affect people of all ages, there are some differences in how it presents and is managed in children versus adults. In children, eczema often appears on the face, scalp, and outer limbs, while adults may experience it more on the hands, feet, and flexural areas (inner elbows and knees). Treatment approaches may also vary based on age and the severity of symptoms.

Common Misconceptions

There are several misconceptions about eczema, including:

- **It's contagious:** Eczema is not contagious and cannot be spread from person to person.

- **It's caused by poor hygiene:** While good hygiene is important, eczema is primarily a genetic and immune-related condition.

- **It's just dry skin:** While dry skin is a symptom, eczema involves inflammation and immune responses that go beyond simple dryness.

- **It can be cured:** While eczema can be managed effectively, there is currently no cure. Treatment focuses on controlling symptoms and preventing flare-ups.

Historical Perspectives

Eczema has been recognized for centuries, with historical references dating back to ancient civilizations. Early treatments often involved topical applications of oils, herbs, and minerals. The understanding of eczema has evolved, leading to more targeted and effective treatments based on scientific research and advancements in dermatology.

Current Research and Developments

Ongoing research in eczema focuses on understanding its underlying mechanisms, developing new treatments, and improving existing therapies. Areas of interest include:

- Identifying genetic factors that contribute to eczema

- Investigating the role of the skin microbiome in eczema development

- Developing targeted immunotherapies and biologics

- Exploring novel topical treatments and formulations

- Studying the impact of lifestyle factors, such as diet and stress, on eczema management

Global Prevalence

Eczema is a global health concern, affecting people of all ages, races, and geographic regions. Its prevalence varies widely depending on factors such as climate, genetics, and environmental exposures. While exact numbers can be challenging to determine due to underreporting and misdiagnosis, eczema is estimated to affect millions of individuals worldwide, highlighting the need for continued research, education, and access to effective treatments.

CHAPTER 2

ANATOMY OF HEALTHY SKIN

Layers of the Skin:

The skin is made up of three primary layers: the epidermis, dermis, and hypodermis. The epidermis is the outermost layer and acts as a protective barrier against external elements. It consists mainly of keratinocytes, which produce the protein keratin that provides structural strength.

Beneath the epidermis lies the dermis, which contains blood vessels, nerves, sweat glands, and hair follicles. It also houses collagen and elastin fibers, which maintain skin elasticity and strength.

The deepest layer is the hypodermis, composed of fat cells (adipocytes) that provide insulation and cushioning for the skin and underlying structures.

Skin Functions:

1. **Protection:** The skin acts as a barrier, protecting the body from harmful microorganisms, UV radiation, and physical injuries.

2. **Temperature Regulation:** Blood vessels in the skin help regulate body temperature by dilating to release heat or constricting to conserve heat.

3. **Sensation:** Nerve endings in the skin allow us to sense touch, pressure, temperature, and pain.

4. **Excretion:** Sweat glands help eliminate waste products and regulate body temperature.

5. **Absorption:** Some substances can be absorbed through the skin, such as medications or certain chemicals.

6. **Synthesis:** The skin synthesizes vitamin D when exposed to sunlight, essential for bone health.

Skin Barrier and Moisture Balance:

The skin barrier is crucial for maintaining hydration and protecting against pathogens. It consists of lipids, ceramides, and proteins that prevent water loss and maintain moisture balance. Disruption of this barrier, as seen in conditions like eczema, can lead to dryness, itching, and increased susceptibility to infections.

Immune Response in the Skin:

The skin has its immune system, with specialized cells like Langerhans cells and T cells that defend against pathogens. Inflammatory responses, such as redness and swelling, are part of the immune reaction to infections or irritants.

Role of Genetics:

Genetics plays a significant role in skin health and susceptibility to conditions like eczema. Certain gene variations can influence skin structure, moisture retention, and immune responses, impacting overall skin resilience.

Environmental Influences:

Factors like UV radiation, pollution, climate, and skincare products can affect skin health. UV exposure, for instance, can lead to premature aging and skin damage, while pollution can trigger inflammation and oxidative stress.

Aging and Skin Changes:

As we age, the skin undergoes various changes, including reduced collagen and elastin production, thinning, and decreased moisture retention. These changes contribute to wrinkles, sagging, and a loss of skin elasticity.

Skin Microbiome:

The skin is home to a diverse microbiome consisting of bacteria, fungi, and other microorganisms. This microbiome plays a role in maintaining skin health by competing with harmful pathogens and supporting immune function.

Skin Health Maintenance:

To maintain healthy skin, it's essential to follow a skincare routine that includes cleansing, moisturizing, sun protection, and avoiding harsh chemicals or irritants. Adequate hydration, a balanced diet rich in antioxidants, and regular exercise also contribute to skin health.

Impact of Lifestyle Choices:

Lifestyle choices such as diet, stress management, sleep quality, and smoking can impact skin health. A balanced diet with vitamins, minerals, and antioxidants supports skin repair and regeneration, while stress and lack of sleep can contribute to skin issues like acne or eczema.

Understanding these aspects of skin anatomy, functions, and maintenance is crucial for promoting healthy skin and managing conditions like eczema effectively.

CHAPTER 3

TRIGGERS AND RISK FACTORS

**Allergens and Irritants:

- Allergens are substances that trigger an allergic reaction, such as pollen, pet dander, dust mites, or certain foods. Irritants, on the other hand, can cause skin irritation or flare-ups without an allergic reaction, like harsh soaps, detergents, or chemicals.

- Identifying and avoiding specific allergens and irritants is crucial in managing eczema. This may involve allergen testing, using hypoallergenic products, and creating an allergen-free environment at home.

Weather Conditions

- Weather can significantly impact eczema, with cold, dry air in winter and hot, humid weather in summer often triggering flare-ups. Rapid changes in temperature and low humidity levels can also worsen symptoms.

- Managing eczema during different seasons may require adjustments to skincare routines, such as using moisturizers more frequently in winter or avoiding excessive sweating in summer.

Stress and Emotional Triggers

- Stress and strong emotions can exacerbate eczema symptoms through the release of stress hormones, which can weaken the skin barrier and increase inflammation.

- Practicing stress management techniques such as mindfulness, meditation, exercise, and seeking support from friends, family, or a therapist can help reduce emotional triggers.

Diet and Nutrition

- Certain foods like dairy, eggs, wheat, soy, and nuts can trigger eczema flare-ups in some individuals. However, food triggers can vary widely from person to person.

- Keeping a food diary, undergoing allergy testing, and working with a healthcare professional or dietitian can help identify and manage dietary triggers

Clothing and Textiles

- Wearing rough, scratchy fabrics like wool or synthetic materials can irritate eczema-prone skin. Tight clothing and clothing with seams or tags can also cause discomfort.

- Opting for soft, breathable fabrics like cotton and using fragrance-free laundry detergents can minimize irritation.

Household Products

- Many household products, including cleaning agents, air fresheners, and personal care products, contain chemicals that can irritate sensitive skin.

- Choosing fragrance-free, hypoallergenic products and minimizing exposure to harsh chemicals can reduce eczema triggers at home.

Medications and Chemicals

- Some medications, particularly topical corticosteroids, and certain antibiotics can cause skin reactions or worsen eczema symptoms in some individuals.

- It's essential to inform healthcare providers about eczema when prescribed medications and to be cautious with over-the-counter products.

Hormonal Influences

- Hormonal changes, such as during puberty, pregnancy, or menopause, can affect eczema severity due to fluctuations in hormone levels.

- Adjusting skincare routines and consulting healthcare providers for hormonal management strategies can help mitigate these effects.

Occupational Factors

- Certain occupations involving frequent hand washing, exposure to chemicals, or working in dry or humid environments can contribute to eczema flare-ups.

- Using protective gloves, moisturizing regularly, and implementing workplace accommodations can minimize occupational triggers.

Identifying Personal Triggers

- Each person with eczema may have unique triggers, making it essential to identify and avoid individualized triggers.

- Keeping a trigger diary, seeking medical advice, and experimenting with lifestyle changes can help pinpoint personal triggers and develop effective management strategies.

Understanding these triggers and risk factors is crucial in managing eczema effectively. Working closely with healthcare professionals, maintaining a consistent skincare routine, and adopting healthy lifestyle habits can significantly improve eczema symptoms and quality of life.

CHAPTER 4

ECZEMA TREATMENTS: FROM CONVENTIONAL TO ALTERNATIVE

Topical Steroids and Moisturizers

- **Topical Steroids**: These are the most common medications prescribed for eczema. They work by reducing inflammation and itching. They are available in various strengths, and your doctor will determine the appropriate one for your condition.

- **Moisturizers**: These are essential for managing eczema as they help keep the skin hydrated and prevent flare-ups. Look for moisturizers that are fragrance-free and hypoallergenic.

Immunomodulators and Biologics

-     **Immunomodulators**:   These are medications that help regulate the immune system's response, reducing inflammation. They are often used when topical steroids are not effective or suitable.

- **Biologics**: These are newer treatments that target specific parts of the immune system involved in eczema. They are usually reserved for severe cases that haven't responded to other treatments.

Antihistamines and Anti-itch Medications

- **Antihistamines**: These can help relieve itching associated with eczema by blocking histamine receptors. They are often used at night to improve sleep quality.

-     **Anti-itch Medications**: Creams or ointments containing ingredients like menthol or pramoxine can provide temporary relief from itching.

Wet Wrap Therapy

- **Wet Wrap Therapy**: This involves applying a moisturizer or medication to the skin, followed by wet bandages. The bandages help lock in moisture and increase the effectiveness of the treatment.

Phototherapy and Light Therapy

- **Phototherapy**: Also known as light therapy, this treatment involves exposing the skin to ultraviolet (UV) light under controlled conditions. It can help reduce inflammation and itching.

- **Light Therapy**: Some devices use specific wavelengths of light, such as narrow-band UVB, which are effective for treating eczema.

Natural Remedies and Home Treatments

- **Natural Remedies**: These may include coconut oil, oatmeal baths, or aloe vera gel, which can provide relief for some people. However, it's essential to consult with a healthcare professional before trying any natural remedies.

- **Home Treatments**: Practices like keeping the skin moisturized, avoiding triggers like harsh soaps or allergens, and maintaining a healthy diet can also help manage eczema.

Dietary Changes and Supplements

- **Dietary Changes**: Some individuals find that certain foods can trigger eczema flare-ups. Keeping a food diary and working with a healthcare provider can help identify and avoid these triggers.

- **Supplements**: Omega-3 fatty acids, probiotics, and vitamin D supplements are among those that may be beneficial for eczema management. However, their effectiveness can vary from person to person.

Acupuncture and Traditional Medicine

- **Acupuncture**: This traditional Chinese medicine practice involves inserting thin needles into specific points on the body to stimulate energy flow and promote healing. Some people with eczema find acupuncture helpful in reducing symptoms.

- **Traditional Medicine**: Herbal remedies and traditional healing practices from various cultures may offer alternative options for managing eczema. It's crucial to consult with trained practitioners for safe and effective treatments.

Psychological Therapies

- **Psychological Support**: Living with eczema can be challenging, especially if it affects your self-esteem or mental well-being. Counseling, support groups, and stress management techniques can help improve overall quality of life.

- **Mindfulness and Relaxation Techniques**: Practices like meditation, deep breathing exercises, and yoga can also be beneficial in reducing stress and managing eczema symptoms.

Integrative Approaches

- **Holistic Care**: Integrative medicine combines conventional treatments with complementary therapies to address the whole person, including physical, emotional, and spiritual aspects.

- **Collaborative Care**: Working with a team of healthcare providers, including dermatologists, allergists, nutritionists, and mental health professionals, can provide comprehensive support for eczema management.

Each of these approaches has its benefits and considerations, and what works best can vary from person to person. It's essential to work closely with healthcare providers to develop a personalized treatment plan that addresses your unique needs and preferences while considering the safety and effectiveness of each method.

CHAPTER 5

MANAGING ECZEMA FLARES

Recognizing Early Signs of Flares

Recognizing the early signs of eczema flares is crucial for effective management. These signs may include increased itching, redness, dryness, or the appearance of small bumps or blisters on the skin. Paying attention to these signals can help you intervene early and prevent the flare from worsening.

Immediate Care Strategies

When a flare occurs, immediate care strategies can provide relief and prevent further aggravation. These strategies may include applying cold compresses to soothe itching, using mild, fragrance-free moisturizers to keep the skin hydrated, and avoiding scratching to prevent skin damage and infection.

Avoiding Triggers

Identifying and avoiding triggers that can exacerbate eczema flares is key to long-term management. Common triggers include certain fabrics, harsh soaps or detergents, extreme temperatures, and stress. By minimizing exposure to these triggers, you can reduce the frequency and severity of flare-ups.

Stress Management Techniques

Stress can significantly impact eczema, triggering flare-ups or making existing ones worse. Incorporating stress management techniques such as mindfulness, deep breathing exercises, regular physical activity, and seeking support from loved ones or mental health professionals can help manage stress and improve eczema outcomes.

Skin Care During Flares

During eczema flares, gentle skin care is paramount. Use mild, non-irritating cleansers and moisturizers specifically designed for sensitive skin. Avoid hot baths or showers, as they can further dry out the skin, and opt for lukewarm water instead. Pat the skin dry gently and apply moisturizer immediately after bathing to lock in moisture.

Adjusting Medications

In some cases, adjusting medications may be necessary to control eczema flares. This may involve topical corticosteroids or other prescribed medications to reduce inflammation and itching. Always follow your healthcare provider's instructions regarding medication use and consult them if you experience any concerns or side effects.

Working with Healthcare Providers

Collaborating closely with healthcare providers is essential for effective eczema management. Your dermatologist or primary care physician can help develop a personalized treatment plan, monitor your progress, and make adjustments as needed. Be sure to communicate openly about your symptoms, concerns, and treatment preferences.

Emergency Preparedness

Having an emergency plan in place is important for handling severe eczema flares or unexpected complications. This plan may include knowing when to seek immediate medical attention, having prescribed medications readily available, and having contact information for healthcare providers easily accessible.

Family and Social Support

Family and social support play a significant role in managing eczema. Educate your loved ones about eczema, its triggers, and how they can support you during flares. Encourage open communication and seek understanding from friends, family, and colleagues to reduce stress and improve overall well-being.

Long-term Flare Prevention

Long-term flare prevention involves a combination of lifestyle modifications, consistent skincare routines, stress management, and regular follow-ups with healthcare providers. By identifying and addressing triggers, maintaining good skincare habits, and staying proactive in managing stress, you can reduce the frequency and severity of eczema flares over time.

Taking a comprehensive approach to managing eczema flares can significantly improve the quality of life and reduce the impact of this chronic skin condition. Regular communication with healthcare providers, self-care practices, and a supportive environment are key components of successful eczema management.

CHAPTER 6

ECZEMA AND QUALITY OF LIFE

Impact on Daily Activities

Eczema can significantly impact daily activities due to its physical symptoms such as itchiness, redness, and inflammation. These symptoms can cause discomfort and affect one's ability to perform routine tasks comfortably. For example, someone with eczema on their hands may find it challenging to do simple activities like cooking, cleaning, or typing. Moreover, the need to constantly manage and treat eczema can consume a significant amount of time and energy, further affecting daily activities.

Sleep Disturbances and Fatigue

Sleep disturbances are common among individuals with eczema, primarily due to the intense itching and discomfort that can worsen at night. Constant scratching can disrupt sleep patterns, leading to fatigue and reduced overall well-being. Lack of quality sleep can also contribute to irritability, difficulty concentrating, and decreased productivity during the day.

Social and Emotional Challenges

Living with eczema can bring about various social and emotional challenges. Visible skin symptoms may lead to self-consciousness, low self-esteem, and feelings of embarrassment or shame. Individuals with eczema may also experience social stigma or discrimination, impacting their social interactions and relationships. Coping with these challenges requires resilience and support from loved ones or professional counselors.

School and Work Accommodations

Eczema may necessitate accommodations at school or work to ensure optimal functioning and well-being. This could include flexible schedules for medical appointments, access to hypoallergenic products, or adjustments in physical environments to minimize triggers that exacerbate eczema symptoms. Open communication with educators or employers about eczema-related needs is essential for creating supportive environments.

Relationships and Intimacy

Eczema can influence relationships and intimacy due to its physical and emotional effects. Partners, family members, or friends may need to understand and accommodate the challenges associated with eczema, such as the need for gentle touch, avoidance of certain fabrics or products, and emotional support during flare-ups. Open communication and empathy are crucial in maintaining healthy relationships and intimacy.

Mental Health Considerations

Living with eczema can impact mental health, leading to stress, anxiety, depression, or other mental health conditions. The chronic nature of eczema, coupled with its visible symptoms and potential social challenges, can contribute to psychological distress. Seeking professional mental health support, practicing stress-reduction techniques, and engaging in self-care activities are essential for managing mental well-being.

Coping Mechanisms

Effective coping mechanisms are vital for individuals with eczema to manage the physical, emotional, and social aspects of the condition. This may include developing a skincare routine with gentle products, practicing stress management techniques like mindfulness or relaxation exercises, seeking social support from peers or support groups, and engaging in enjoyable activities that promote overall well-being.

Advocacy and Support Groups

Advocacy and support groups play a crucial role in empowering individuals with eczema and advocating for their needs. These groups provide a platform for sharing experiences, accessing resources, raising awareness about eczema-related issues, and advocating for policy changes or research funding. Engaging with advocacy organizations and support groups can foster a sense of community and empowerment.

Educational Resources

Access to reliable educational resources is essential for individuals with eczema, their caregivers, and healthcare providers. These resources may include websites, publications, workshops, or educational materials that offer information about eczema management, treatment options, lifestyle modifications, and coping strategies. Staying informed and educated empowers individuals to make informed decisions about their health.

Enhancing Quality of Life

Enhancing quality of life for individuals with eczema involves a holistic approach that addresses physical, emotional, and social well-being. This includes effective symptom management, adopting healthy lifestyle habits, fostering supportive relationships, seeking professional support when needed, participating in advocacy efforts, and engaging in activities that promote joy and fulfillment.

By addressing these aspects comprehensively, individuals with eczema can improve their overall quality of life and well-being.

CHAPTER 7

SKINCARE AND MAINTENANCE ROUTINE

Gentle Cleansing Techniques:

- **Frequency**: Aim for bathing or showering once daily or every other day to avoid over-drying the skin.

- **Water Temperature**: Use lukewarm water instead of hot water, as hot water can strip the skin of natural oils.

- **Cleanser Selection**: Opt for mild, fragrance-free cleansers formulated for sensitive skin or specifically for eczema.

- **Application**: Gently lather the cleanser on your hands before applying it to your skin, and avoid harsh scrubbing or rubbing.

Moisturizing Practices:

- **Timing**: Apply moisturizer immediately after bathing or showering to lock in moisture.

- **Type of Moisturizer**: Choose thick, ointment-based moisturizers or creams rather than lotions, as they provide better hydration.

- **Frequency**: Reapply moisturizer throughout the day as needed, especially in dry or cold environments.

- **Ingredients**: Look for moisturizers containing ceramides, hyaluronic acid, and shea butter, which help repair and protect the skin barrier.

Bathing and Showering Tips:

- **Avoiding Harsh Soaps**: Use gentle, fragrance-free soaps or cleansers formulated for sensitive skin.

- **Shorter Showers**: Limit shower or bath time to 10-15 minutes to prevent excessive drying of the skin.

- **Pat Dry**: Gently pat your skin dry with a soft towel instead of rubbing vigorously.

- **Moisturize Immediately**: Apply moisturizer within 3 minutes of leaving the shower or bath to seal in moisture.

Clothing Selection:

- **Fabric Choice**: Wear loose-fitting, breathable clothing made from soft fabrics like cotton or silk.

- **Avoid Irritants**: Wash new clothes before wearing them to remove any potential irritants or chemicals.

- **Weather Consideration**: In colder weather, layer clothing to avoid overheating and sweating, which can exacerbate eczema.

Avoiding Skin Irritants:

- **Fragrances and Dyes**: Choose skin care products, detergents, and household cleaners labeled "fragrance-free" and "dye-free."

- **Harsh Chemicals**: Avoid products containing alcohol, parabens, sulfates, and other harsh chemicals that can irritate sensitive skin.

- **Patch Testing**: Before trying new products, perform a patch test on a small area of skin to check for reactions.

Sun Protection:

- **Sunscreen**: Use a broad-spectrum sunscreen with an SPF of 30 or higher, and reapply every 2 hours when outdoors.

- **Protective Clothing**: Wear wide-brimmed hats, long sleeves, and pants to shield your skin from the sun.

- **Seek Shade**: Limit sun exposure, especially during peak sunlight hours from 10 am to 4 pm.

Nail and Hair Care:

- **Nail Trimming**: Keep your nails short and clean to reduce the risk of scratching and causing skin damage.

- **Gloves**: Wear gloves when doing tasks that may irritate your skin, such as washing dishes or gardening.

- **Hair Care Products**: Choose gentle, hypoallergenic shampoos and conditioners without harsh chemicals or fragrances.

Sleep Environment:

- **Bedding Materials**: Use hypoallergenic bedding, including pillows and mattress covers, to reduce exposure to allergens.

- **Humidity Control**: Maintain a comfortable humidity level in your bedroom, as dry air can worsen eczema symptoms.

- **Cool Temperatures**: Keep your bedroom cool to prevent overheating during sleep, which can trigger itching.

Exercise and Sweat Management:

- **Clothing Choice**: Wear moisture-wicking fabrics during exercise to help manage sweat and prevent skin irritation.

- **Shower After Exercise**: Rinse off sweat and promptly shower after exercising to remove potential irritants from your skin.

- **Hydration**: Drink plenty of water to stay hydrated, which can improve overall skin health.

Regular Monitoring and Check-ups:

- **Skin Self-Exams**: Regularly inspect your skin for any changes, such as new rashes, redness, or irritation.

- **Dermatologist Visits**: Schedule regular check-ups with your dermatologist to monitor your eczema and adjust your treatment plan as needed.

- **Medication Adherence**: Follow your dermatologist's prescribed medications and treatments consistently to manage eczema flare-ups effectively.

By incorporating these skincare and maintenance practices into your daily routine, you can help manage eczema symptoms and promote healthier, more comfortable skin. It's essential to be patient and consistent with these strategies, as eczema management often requires ongoing care and attention.

CHAPTER 8

ECZEMA IN SPECIAL POPULATIONS

Pediatric Eczema: Challenges and Treatments

Pediatric eczema presents unique challenges due to the delicate nature of a child's skin and their limited ability to communicate discomfort. It often manifests as itchy, red patches that can be distressing for both the child and their caregivers. Treatment involves gentle skincare routines, avoiding triggers like harsh soaps or allergens, and using moisturizers and topical corticosteroids as prescribed by a pediatrician or dermatologist. Education for parents on how to manage flare-ups and prevent skin infections is crucial.

Eczema in Elderly Individuals

Eczema in older adults can be exacerbated by age-related changes in the skin, such as reduced moisture retention and thinning. It may also coincide with other skin conditions or medical issues. Treatment focuses on hydrating the skin, using emollients, and addressing any underlying factors like allergies or immune system changes. Regular monitoring by a healthcare professional is essential to manage eczema effectively in this population.

Pregnancy and Eczema

Pregnancy can impact eczema, with some women experiencing flare-ups due to hormonal changes or stress. However, certain treatments may need to be adjusted to ensure safety for both the mother and the developing baby. Emollients and mild topical corticosteroids are generally considered safe during pregnancy, but it's crucial to consult with a healthcare provider for personalized recommendations.

Eczema in Athletes

Athletes with eczema face unique challenges due to increased sweat, friction from clothing or equipment, and exposure to potential triggers like chlorine in pools. Proper skincare before and after activities, choosing breathable fabrics, and showering immediately after sweating can help manage eczema in athletes. Dermatologist guidance may be necessary for severe cases or if eczema impacts athletic performance.

Managing Eczema in Different Seasons

Eczema can fluctuate with seasonal changes, with winter often exacerbating symptoms due to dry indoor air and cold weather. Summer may present challenges with increased heat and sun exposure. Adjusting skincare routines, using humidifiers in winter, and applying sunscreen in summer are strategies to manage eczema across seasons. Personalized care plans based on seasonal triggers are beneficial.

Eczema in People with Compromised Immunity

Individuals with compromised immune systems, such as those with HIV/AIDS or undergoing immunosuppressive therapy, may experience more severe or recurrent eczema. Close monitoring by healthcare professionals is essential to balance eczema management with immune health. Specialized treatments or adjustments in medication may be necessary to address eczema effectively in this population.

Cultural and Ethnic Considerations

Cultural and ethnic factors can influence how eczema is perceived, managed, and treated. For example, certain cultural practices or beliefs may impact skincare routines or access to healthcare services. Healthcare providers should be culturally competent and considerate of these factors when developing eczema management plans, ensuring inclusivity and effective communication.

LGBTQ+ Community and Eczema

Eczema can affect individuals within the LGBTQ+ community, and their experiences may be influenced by various factors, including hormone therapy, stress related to identity, or specific healthcare needs. Providing a supportive and inclusive environment in healthcare settings is crucial for LGBTQ+ individuals with eczema to receive personalized care and feel comfortable discussing their concerns.

Eczema and Chronic Illnesses

Eczema often coexists with other chronic illnesses like asthma or allergies, leading to complex management needs. Healthcare providers should consider comorbidities and potential interactions when developing treatment plans. Collaboration between specialists may be necessary to address all aspects of a patient's health effectively.

Addressing Unique Needs

Each individual with eczema has unique needs based on factors such as age, lifestyle, coexisting conditions, and personal preferences. Tailoring treatment plans to address these specific needs ensures optimal outcomes. Regular follow-ups, patient education, and ongoing support are essential components of holistic eczema care.

These topics highlight the diverse considerations and approaches required to effectively manage eczema in special populations, emphasizing the importance of personalized care, education, and collaboration among healthcare providers and patients.

CHAPTER 9

EMERGING TRENDS AND INNOVATIONS

Advances in Eczema Research:

Eczema research has seen significant strides in recent years, focusing on understanding the underlying causes and mechanisms of the condition. Scientists are delving into genetics, immunology, and environmental factors to unravel the complexities of eczema. Cutting-edge technologies like genomics and proteomics are aiding researchers in identifying specific biomarkers associated with different types of eczema, leading to more targeted treatments.

Precision Medicine and Personalized Treatments:

The advent of precision medicine has revolutionized eczema treatment by tailoring therapies to individual patients based on their genetic makeup, immune responses, and environmental triggers. This approach not only enhances treatment efficacy but also reduces adverse effects by avoiding one-size-fits-all strategies. Personalized treatments may include targeted biologics, immunomodulators, or allergen-specific therapies, offering hope for better outcomes and improved quality of life for eczema patients.

Novel Therapies in Development:

Innovative therapies are emerging in the field of eczema, ranging from topical formulations to biological agents and gene therapies. Topical treatments with novel drug delivery systems are designed for enhanced skin penetration and prolonged efficacy. Biologics targeting specific immune pathways are undergoing clinical trials, showing promising results in severe eczema cases. Gene editing techniques like CRISPR offer potential long-term solutions by correcting genetic mutations associated with eczema.

Technology in Eczema Management:

Technology plays a pivotal role in modern eczema management, offering tools for tracking symptoms, monitoring flare-ups, and improving patient adherence to treatment regimens. Mobile apps and wearable devices provide real-time data on skin conditions, environmental triggers, and medication schedules, empowering patients and healthcare providers with valuable insights for personalized care.

Artificial Intelligence in Healthcare:

Artificial intelligence (AI) is revolutionizing healthcare, including eczema management, by analyzing vast amounts of data to predict disease progression, optimize treatment plans, and enhance diagnostic accuracy. AI-powered algorithms can identify patterns in eczema triggers, predict flare-ups, and recommend personalized interventions, improving outcomes and reducing healthcare costs.

Telemedicine and Virtual Care

Telemedicine has become increasingly popular in eczema care, enabling remote consultations, virtual follow-ups, and easy access to specialists. This approach improves patient convenience, reduces travel burdens, and ensures timely interventions, especially in rural or underserved areas. Virtual care platforms integrate video consultations, secure messaging, and electronic health records, facilitating seamless communication between patients and providers.

Patient-Provider Communication Tools

Effective communication between patients and healthcare providers is essential for managing eczema effectively. Digital communication tools such as secure messaging platforms, patient portals, and virtual support groups promote ongoing dialogue, shared decision-making, and collaborative care plans. These tools foster trust, enhance treatment adherence, and empower patients to take an active role in their eczema management.

Wearable Devices for Skin Monitoring

Wearable devices equipped with sensors and biometric technology enable continuous monitoring of skin parameters such as moisture levels, temperature, and inflammation markers. These devices provide real-time feedback, alerting patients to potential triggers and helping healthcare providers monitor treatment responses remotely. Wearable technology enhances self-management strategies and promotes early intervention for better eczema control.

Environmental Sustainability in Eczema Products

The shift towards environmentally sustainable practices in eczema products reflects a growing awareness of ecological impacts and consumer preferences. Companies are developing eco-friendly formulations using renewable resources, recyclable packaging, and biodegradable materials. Sustainable practices not only benefit the environment but also promote skin health by minimizing exposure to harmful chemicals and irritants.

Future Outlook and Expectations

The future of eczema care holds immense promise with ongoing advancements in research, technology, and personalized medicine. Expectations include more targeted therapies based on individualized profiles, innovative drug delivery systems for improved efficacy, and integrated digital solutions for seamless patient-provider collaboration. Environmental sustainability will continue to shape product development, ensuring safer and greener options for eczema management. Overall, the outlook is optimistic for enhanced outcomes and a better quality of life for eczema patients worldwide.

CHAPTER 10

EMPOWERING YOURSELF AND OTHERS

Self-Advocacy Skills

Empowering yourself through self-advocacy in dealing with eczema involves understanding your condition, its triggers, and treatments. It includes effectively communicating your needs to healthcare providers, asking questions, and seeking second opinions when necessary. Self-advocacy also entails staying informed about new research and treatment options, advocating for yourself in insurance matters, and being proactive in managing your health.

Building a Support Network

Building a support network is crucial for individuals with eczema. This network can include healthcare professionals, family members, friends, support groups, and online communities. Having a support network provides emotional support, practical advice, and a sense of belonging. It can also help in finding resources, sharing experiences, and coping with challenges related to eczema.

Educating Family and Friends

Educating family and friends about eczema is essential for creating a supportive environment. This involves explaining the condition, its symptoms, triggers, and treatment options. It also includes discussing the impact of eczema on daily life, such as skin care routines, dietary considerations, and emotional well-being. Educating loved ones helps foster understanding, empathy, and effective support.

Navigating Healthcare Systems

Navigating healthcare systems can be complex, but it's necessary for managing eczema effectively. This includes understanding health insurance coverage, finding knowledgeable healthcare providers, scheduling appointments, and accessing medications and treatments. It also involves advocating for comprehensive care, including dermatology, allergy testing, and mental health support if needed.

Participating in Research and Clinical Trials

Participating in research and clinical trials contributes to advancing knowledge and improving treatments for eczema. It offers individuals the opportunity to access cutting-edge therapies, contribute to scientific discoveries, and connect with experts in the field. Before participating, individuals should carefully consider risks, benefits, and eligibility criteria, and consult with healthcare providers.

Community Engagement and Volunteering

Engaging with the eczema community through volunteering, advocacy, or support groups can be empowering and fulfilling. It allows individuals to connect with others facing similar challenges, share experiences, and make a positive impact. Community engagement also raises awareness, promotes education, and advocates for improved access to care and resources.

Raising Awareness

Raising awareness about eczema is essential for promoting understanding, reducing stigma, and advocating for better support and resources. This can be done through public campaigns, educational events, social media, and personal storytelling. Raising awareness helps educate the public, healthcare providers, policymakers, and communities about eczema's impact and the needs of those affected.

Overcoming Stigma and Misconceptions

Overcoming stigma and misconceptions surrounding eczema involves challenging stereotypes, promoting accurate information, and advocating for acceptance and inclusion. This includes addressing myths about the condition, educating others about its physical and emotional aspects, and emphasizing the importance of empathy and support. Overcoming stigma helps individuals with eczema feel validated, respected, and understood.

Mentorship and Peer Support

Mentorship and peer support play a significant role in empowering individuals with eczema. Mentors can provide guidance, encouragement, and practical advice based on their experiences. Peer support groups offer a sense of community, shared understanding, and mutual support. Both mentorship and peer support foster resilience, confidence, and personal growth.

Inspiring Stories of Triumph

Sharing inspiring stories of triumph can motivate and uplift individuals with eczema. These stories highlight resilience, perseverance, and the ability to thrive despite challenges. They offer hope, encouragement, and a sense of solidarity. Inspiring stories also showcase diverse experiences and strategies for managing eczema, inspiring others to take control of their health and well-being.